THE NATURAL WAY TO HEAL STOMACH ULCERS

Proven Diet and Lifestyle Changes for Ulcer Relief

Kayla S. Brigman

Kayla S. Brigman

Library of Congress Cataloging-in-Publication Data

Brigman, Kayla S.

The Natural Way to Heal Stomach Ulcers: Proven Diet and Lifestyle Changes for Ulcer Relief

Year of Publication: 2023

ISBN-13: 9798386563585

Printed in the United States of America

Cover design by *Louis J. Baltz*

Interior design by *Arlene van Roosmalen*

Dedication

This book is dedicated to all those who have suffered the pain and discomfort of stomach ulcers. May the natural strategies and proven techniques within these pages bring you lasting relief and renewed hope for a healthier future.

Foreword

As a medical doctor with decades of experience in the field of gastroenterology, I have seen firsthand the devastating effects that stomach ulcers can have on a person's health and quality of life. For years, the standard approach to treating stomach ulcers involved a combination of medication and lifestyle changes, with varying degrees of success.

However, as our understanding of the human body and its complex interplay with the environment has evolved, so too has our approach to healing. In recent years, there has been a growing recognition of the power of natural remedies and holistic therapies to complement and enhance traditional medical treatments.

That is why I am so excited to introduce *"The Natural Way to Heal Stomach Ulcers"* by Kayla S. Brigman. This book provides a comprehensive guide to natural strategies and proven techniques that can help alleviate the symptoms of stomach ulcers and promote long-term healing.

Drawing on the latest scientific research and his extensive experience as a natural health practitioner, Kayla provides practical advice and actionable steps that readers can take to address the root causes of their stomach ulcers and achieve lasting relief. From dietary changes to herbal remedies to stress-reducing techniques, this book covers a wide range of natural approaches that can help optimize your health and well-being.

I believe that this book has the potential to revolutionize the way we approach the treatment of stomach ulcers. By embracing the power of natural healing and taking an integrative approach to health, we can achieve better outcomes for ourselves and our patients.

I wholeheartedly recommend "*The Natural Way to Heal Stomach Ulcers*" to anyone who is seeking a holistic, natural approach to healing and well-being.

Walter S. McQuillen, MD

Table of Contents

Introduction

If you're suffering from stomach ulcers, you know firsthand how painful and disruptive they can be. You may have tried traditional treatments, such as medications and surgery, but they only provided temporary relief or had undesirable side effects.

If you're looking for a more holistic approach to healing, you're in the right place. This book is designed to provide a comprehensive understanding of stomach ulcers and offer practical, natural strategies for relieving and preventing them.

We'll start by exploring the causes and symptoms of stomach ulcers, as well as the risks associated with them. From there, we'll delve into various natural remedies and lifestyle changes that can help heal and prevent ulcers. These include dietary changes, stress management techniques, and herbal remedies.

Throughout the book, you'll find helpful tips, case studies, and resources to guide you to lasting stomach ulcer relief. With the knowledge and strategies provided in this book, you can take control of your health and find relief from the pain and discomfort of stomach ulcers.

So let's get started on your path to healing!

Chapter 1

Introduction to Stomach Ulcers: Causes, Symptoms, and Risks

A stomach ulcer, or peptic ulcer, is a sore in the stomach lining or small intestine. The most common cause of stomach ulcers is the bacterium Helicobacter pylori or H. pylori. These bacteria can damage the protective lining of the stomach, leading to the formation of an ulcer.

Other potential causes of stomach ulcers include nonsteroidal anti-inflammatory drugs (NSAIDs) such as ibuprofen and aspirin and excessive alcohol consumption.

The most common symptom of a stomach ulcer is a burning or gnawing pain in the upper abdomen. This pain may be relieved by eating or taking antacids, but it often returns. Other stomach ulcer symptoms may include nausea, vomiting, weight loss, and bloating.

If left untreated, stomach ulcers can lead to serious health risks. Ulcers can cause bleeding in the digestive tract, which can lead to anaemia and other complications. Ulcers can also cause a perforation, or hole, in the wall of the digestive tract, which can be life-threatening.

Understanding the Role of H. pylori in Stomach Ulcers

H. pylori is a bacterium that infects the stomach lining and small intestine. It is a leading cause of stomach ulcers and is responsible for approximately 50% of all ulcers. H. pylori is transmitted through contaminated food and water, which is more common in areas with poor sanitation.

Infection with H. pylori can cause inflammation and damage to the protective lining of the stomach, leading to the formation of an ulcer. H. pylori infection can also increase the production of stomach acid, which can further irritate the stomach lining and cause ulcer formation.

Treatment for H. pylori-related stomach ulcers typically involves a combination of antibiotics and acid-reducing medications. Natural remedies may also effectively reduce the symptoms of H. pylori infection and help to heal the ulcer. These remedies may include probiotics, herbal remedies, and dietary changes.

In the following chapters, we'll delve into the various natural remedies and lifestyle changes that can help heal and prevent stomach ulcers. But first, it's essential to understand the role that H. pylori can play in developing these sores. By understanding this factor, you can take steps to address the root cause of your ulcer and find lasting relief.

The Power of Stress Reduction for Stomach Ulcer Healing

Stress is a fact of life, but when it comes to stomach ulcers, it can be a significant trigger for symptoms. When you are under stress, your body produces cortisol, a hormone that can increase acid production in your stomach and worsen your ulcer symptoms. This section will explore the relationship between stress and stomach ulcers and provide practical guidance on reducing stress to promote healing.

The Link between Stress and Stomach Ulcers

While stress does not directly cause stomach ulcers, it can worsen them. When you are under pressure, your body produces more acid in the stomach, leading to irritation and inflammation of the stomach lining. This can trigger symptoms like abdominal pain, bloating, nausea, and indigestion.

Chronic stress can also weaken your immune system, making it harder for your body to fight infections like H. pylori. These bacteria are often responsible for causing stomach ulcers.

Stress Reduction Techniques for Stomach Ulcer Healing

Reducing stress is an essential part of managing stomach ulcers. Here are some stress reduction techniques that can help to promote healing:

1. *Mindfulness meditation:*

Focusing on the present moment while accepting your thoughts and emotions without judgment is part of the mindfulness meditation approach. It has been shown to lessen stress and anxiety while enhancing general well-being.

2. *Yoga:*

Yoga is a physical and mental practice that combines breath control, meditation, and physical postures. It has been shown to reduce stress and improve mood.

3. *Deep breathing exercises:*

Deep breathing exercises can help to calm your nervous system and reduce stress. Try taking slow, deep breaths through your nose and out through your mouth for a few minutes each day.

4. *Exercise:*

Exercise is a natural stress reducer that can promote healing by increasing blood flow to your stomach and reducing inflammation.

5. *Social support:*

Talking to friends and family members can help reduce stress and provide support and connection.

The Bottom Line

Stress can worsen stomach ulcer symptoms, but there are many effective techniques for reducing stress and promoting healing. Mindfulness meditation, yoga, deep breathing exercises, exercise, and social support effectively reduce stress and improve overall well-being.

By incorporating these techniques into your daily routine, you can take control of your stress levels and promote lasting relief from stomach ulcers.

In the next chapter, we'll delve into the importance of a healthy diet in stomach ulcer healing. By understanding these factors, you can take control of your health and find relief from the pain and discomfort of stomach ulcers.

Chapter 2

The Importance of a Healthy Diet in Stomach Ulcer Healing

Diet plays a significant role in the health of your digestive system and can significantly impact the healing and prevention of stomach ulcers. Certain foods and drinks can irritate the lining of the stomach and increase the risk of ulcer formation, while others can help heal and prevent ulcers.

Foods to avoid if you have or are at risk for stomach ulcers include:

- Alcohol

- Caffeine

- Spicy foods

- Acidic foods (such as citrus fruits)

- Processed meats (such as deli meat and bacon)

- Fried foods

On the other hand, several foods may be helpful in healing and preventing stomach ulcers. These include:

- Fruits and vegetables, which are rich in antioxidants and help to protect the lining of the digestive tract

- Whole grains, which are high in fiber and can help to regulate digestion

- Lean proteins, such as chicken, fish, and tofu, which are easy on the digestive system

- Healthy fats, such as olive oil and avocado, which can help to reduce inflammation and support the healing process

In addition to making dietary changes, it's also essential to maintain a healthy weight, as being overweight or obese can increase the risk of ulcer formation.

It's essential to understand the role that diet plays in the health of your digestive system. By making mindful dietary choices, you can support the healing process and reduce your risk of ulcer formation.

The Role of Stress Management in Stomach Ulcer Healing

Stress is a natural part of life and can significantly impact physical and mental health. Chronic stress can contribute to the development of stomach ulcers and exacerbate existing ulcers' symptoms.

One of the ways that stress can contribute to ulcer formation is by increasing the production of stomach acid. This procedure can irritate the stomach lining and lead to ulcer formation. Stress can also weaken the immune system, making it more difficult for the body to fight off infections such as H. pylori, a leading cause of stomach ulcers.

To manage stress and support the healing and prevention of stomach ulcers, you must adopt stress management strategies that work for you. These may include:

- Exercise, which can help to reduce stress and improve the overall health

- Meditation and mindfulness practices, which can help to calm the mind and reduce stress

- Counseling or therapy, which can provide a safe space to process and manage stress

- Time management techniques, which can help to reduce the feeling of being overwhelmed

- Relaxation techniques, such as deep breathing or progressive muscle relaxation

It's also important to prioritize self-care and make time for activities that bring you joy and relaxation. By managing stress and adopting a healthy lifestyle, you can support the healing and prevention of stomach ulcers and improve your overall health and well-being.

The Role of Nutrition in Stomach Ulcer Healing

If you are suffering from a stomach ulcer, paying close attention to what you eat is crucial. While diet alone cannot cure an ulcer, it can significantly promote healing and prevent future flare-ups. This section will explore the relationship between nutrition and stomach ulcer healing and provide practical guidance on what to eat and avoid.

The Importance of a Healthy Diet for Stomach Ulcer Healing

Your stomach lining is already inflamed and sensitive when you have a stomach ulcer. Eating foods high in acid, spicy, or hard to digest can irritate your stomach further, worsening your symptoms. Conversely, eating a diet rich in whole, nutrient-dense foods can help to soothe inflammation and promote healing.

Foods to Eat for Stomach Ulcer Healing

A diet rich in whole, plant-based foods is the best way to promote healing and reduce inflammation. Here are some specific foods that are especially beneficial for stomach ulcer healing:

1. High-fiber foods:

Fiber-rich foods like fruits, vegetables, legumes, and whole grains can help to regulate digestion, prevent constipation, and support the growth of healthy gut bacteria.

2. Fermented foods:

Fermented foods like kefir, kimchi, sauerkraut, and miso contain probiotics that can help to promote a healthy gut microbiome.

3. Antioxidant-rich foods:

Antioxidants like vitamins C, E, and beta-carotene can help to protect your stomach lining from further damage. Foods like berries, leafy greens, and nuts are excellent sources of antioxidants.

4. *Lean protein:*

Protein is essential for repairing and rebuilding tissue. Opt for lean protein sources like chicken, fish, and tofu, and avoid fatty or processed meats.

5. *Healthy fats:*

Healthy fats like omega-3 fatty acids can help to reduce inflammation in the body. Good sources of healthy fats include seeds, fatty fish, nuts, and avocado.

Foods to Avoid for Stomach Ulcer Healing

Just as there are foods that can promote healing, there are also foods that can irritate your stomach and worsen your symptoms. As someone suffering from stomach ulcer, here are some foods to avoid:

1. *Spicy foods:*

Spices like chili powder, black pepper, and hot sauce can irritate your stomach lining and worsen your symptoms.

2. *Acidic foods:*

Foods high in acid, like citrus fruits, tomatoes, and vinegar, can also irritate your stomach lining.

3. *Fried foods:*

Fried foods are high in fat and can be challenging to digest, worsening your symptoms.

4. *Alcohol and caffeine:*

Both alcohol and caffeine can irritate your stomach lining and increase acid production, worsening your symptoms.

5. Processed foods:

Processed foods are often high in salt, sugar, and unhealthy fats, all of which can contribute to inflammation in the body.

The Bottom Line

While a healthy diet alone cannot cure a stomach ulcer, it can significantly promote healing and prevent future flare-ups. A diet rich in whole, plant-based foods, lean protein, and healthy fats and low in spicy, acidic, and processed foods is the best way to support your stomach ulcer healing journey.

With a little effort and attention, you can take control of your nutrition and promote lasting relief from stomach ulcers.

Chapter 3

Natural Remedies for Stomach Ulcer Relief: Herbs, Spices, and Other Options

You're not alone if you're seeking natural remedies for stomach ulcer relief. Many people turn to natural remedies as an alternative to traditional medications, which can have unwanted side effects.

While natural remedies may not work for everyone, they can be a safe and effective option for some people.

Some natural remedies that may help relieve the symptoms of stomach ulcers include:

- **Herbs:**

Certain herbs, such as licorice root, slippery elm, and marshmallow root, may help to soothe the lining of the stomach and promote healing.

- **Spices:**

Spices such as turmeric and ginger may help to reduce inflammation and promote healing.

- **Acupuncture:**

Acupuncture involves inserting thin needles into the body at specific points. It is a traditional Chinese medicine practice. In addition to reducing pain, it may promote healing as well.

- **Massage therapy:**

Massage therapy may help reduce stress and promote relaxation, which can benefit stomach ulcer healing.

- ***Homeopathy:***

A homeopathic treatment stimulates the body's natural healing processes by using highly diluted substances. Homeopathic remedies for stomach ulcers may include remedies made from plants, minerals, and animal products.

It's important to note that the effectiveness of natural remedies may vary from person to person, and it's always best to consult with a healthcare professional before starting any new treatment.

In the following chapters, we'll delve into the various natural remedies and lifestyle changes that can help heal and prevent stomach ulcers. By incorporating natural remedies into your treatment plan, you can find relief from the pain and discomfort of stomach ulcers and support the healing process.

The Role of Probiotics in Stomach Ulcer Healing and Prevention

Probiotics are beneficial bacteria that live in the digestive system and help maintain a healthy microorganism's balance. There is some evidence to suggest that probiotics may be helpful in the healing and prevention of stomach ulcers.

One of the ways that probiotics may be beneficial is by helping to reduce the population of H. pylori bacteria in the digestive system. H. pylori is a leading cause of stomach ulcers, and reducing the population of these bacteria can help to reduce the risk of ulcer formation. Probiotics may also help reduce digestive system inflammation and promote healing.

Probiotics can be found in fermented foods such as yogurt, kefir, and sauerkraut, as well as in supplements. It's essential to choose a high-quality probiotic supplement and to follow the recommended dosage.

It's also important to note that the effectiveness of probiotics may vary from person to person, and more research is needed to understand their role in stomach ulcer healing and prevention fully. As with any treatment, it's always best to consult a healthcare professional before starting a probiotic regimen.

Natural Remedies for Stomach Ulcers

While medication is often the first line of treatment for stomach ulcers, natural remedies can also promote healing and reduce symptoms. This section will explore some of the most effective natural remedies for stomach ulcers, including herbs, supplements, and home remedies.

Herbs for Stomach Ulcers

Several herbs have been traditionally used to treat stomach ulcers. Some of the most effective herbs for stomach ulcers include the following:

1. *Licorice root:*

Licorice root has anti-inflammatory properties and can help to soothe the stomach lining. It is often used in combination with other herbs for maximum effectiveness.

2. *Ginger:*

Ginger has been shown to reduce inflammation and promote the healing of the stomach lining. It can be taken in capsule form or brewed as tea.

3. *Turmeric:*

Turmeric has anti-inflammatory properties and can help to reduce inflammation in the stomach lining. It can be taken in capsule form or added to food as a spice.

4. *Chamomile:*

Chamomile has anti-inflammatory properties and can help to reduce inflammation in the stomach lining. It can be brewed as tea.

Supplements for Stomach Ulcers

Several supplements are effective in promoting healing and reducing symptoms of stomach ulcers. Some of the most effective supplements for stomach ulcers are as follows:

- **Probiotics**: Probiotics can help to restore the balance of bacteria in the gut and reduce inflammation in the stomach lining.

- **Vitamin C:** Vitamin C is essential for collagen production, which is necessary to heal the stomach lining and also boost the immune system.

- **Zinc:** Zinc is essential for healing the stomach lining and can help reduce inflammation.

Home Remedies for Stomach Ulcers

Several home remedies can effectively reduce symptoms and promote the healing of stomach ulcers. Some of the effective home remedies for curing stomach ulcers are as follows:

- **Aloe vera juice:** Aloe vera juice can help to reduce inflammation in the stomach lining and promote healing. It can be taken as a supplement or added to water or juice.

- **Honey:** Honey has antibacterial properties and can help kill H. pylori, the bacteria often responsible for causing stomach ulcers. It can be taken as a supplement or added to tea or other beverages.

- **Slippery elm**: Slippery elm can help to soothe the stomach lining and reduce inflammation. It can be taken in capsule form or brewed as tea.

The Bottom Line

Natural remedies like herbs, supplements and home remedies can play a role in promoting healing and reducing symptoms of stomach ulcers.

- Herbs like licorice root, ginger, turmeric, and chamomile can effectively reduce inflammation and promote healing.

- Supplements like probiotics, vitamin C, and zinc can also be adequate.

- Home remedies like aloe vera juice, honey, and slippery elm can also help to soothe the stomach lining and reduce inflammation.

However, talking to your doctor before using any natural remedies is essential, as they can interact with other medications and may not be safe for everyone.

In the following chapters, we'll delve into the various natural remedies and lifestyle changes that can help heal and prevent stomach ulcers. Incorporating probiotics into your treatment plan can support the healing process and reduce your risk of ulcer formation.

Chapter 4

Lifestyle Changes for Stomach Ulcer Healing and Prevention

Lifestyle changes can be an essential part of the healing and prevention of stomach ulcers. Making small changes to your daily routine can support the healing process and reduce your risk of ulcer formation.

Here are some lifestyle changes that may be helpful in the healing and prevention of stomach ulcers:

- **Quit smoking:**

Smoking can irritate the stomach lining and increase the risk of ulcer formation. Quitting smoking can help to reduce this risk and support the healing process.

- **Reduce alcohol consumption:**

Excessive alcohol consumption can irritate the stomach lining and increase the risk of ulcer formation. Reducing your alcohol intake can help reduce this risk and support healing.

- **Maintain a healthy weight:**

Being overweight or obese can increase the risk of ulcer formation. Maintaining a healthy weight can reduce this risk and support the healing process.

- **Get enough sleep:**

Poor sleep can contribute to stress and weaken the immune system, increasing the risk of ulcer formation. Getting enough sleep can help reduce this risk and support healing.

- ***Practice stress management techniques:***

Chronic stress can contribute to ulcer formation and exacerbate the symptoms of existing ulcers. Stress management techniques, such as exercise, meditation, and counseling, can help reduce stress and support the healing process.

In the following chapters, we'll delve into the various natural remedies and lifestyle changes that can help heal and prevent stomach ulcers. By making minor changes to your daily routine, you can take control of your health and find relief from the pain and discomfort of stomach ulcers.

The Connection between Stomach Ulcers and Sleep

Sleep is essential to our overall health and well-being, and it plays a vital role in healing and preventing stomach ulcers. Poor sleep can contribute to stress and weaken the immune system, increasing the risk of ulcer formation. On the other hand, getting enough sleep can help to reduce stress, boost the immune system, and support the healing process.

Several factors can impact the quality of our sleep, including:

1. **Stress**: Chronic stress can interfere with the body's sleep cycle and lead to insomnia.

2. **Diet**: A healthy, balanced diet can support the body's natural sleep cycle. On the other hand, consuming caffeine and alcohol close to bedtime can interfere with sleep.

3. ***Sleep environment***: Creating a comfortable, dark, and quiet sleep environment can help to promote restful sleep.

4. ***Sleep habits***: Developing healthy sleep habits, such as going to bed at the same time each night and avoiding screens before bedtime, can help to improve sleep quality.

If you're struggling with sleep, there are several strategies you can try to improve your sleep quality:

- Take time to relax before bedtime by practicing relaxation techniques such as progressive muscle relaxation or deep breathing

- Avoid screens for at least one hour before bedtime

- Create a comfortable sleep environment, including a comfortable bed and pillows

- Establish a consistent sleep schedule

- Avoid alcohol and caffeine close to bedtime

By prioritizing sleep and adopting healthy sleep habits, you can support the healing and prevention of stomach ulcers and improve your overall health and well-being.

Mind-Body Techniques for Healing Stomach Ulcers

Stomach ulcers are a common medical condition that can cause significant discomfort and pain. Ulcers occur when the stomach's protective lining is eroded, leading to open sores that can bleed and cause inflammation.

While medical treatment is essential for healing stomach ulcers, mind-body techniques can also significantly reduce symptoms and promote recovery.

Meditation

Meditation is a popular mind-body technique that involves focusing the mind on a particular thought, object, or activity. This practice has been shown to reduce stress and anxiety, known risk factors for stomach ulcers. Chronic stress can lead to increased acid production in the stomach, which can exacerbate ulcer symptoms.

Meditation has been shown to reduce stress levels, decrease the production of stress hormones, and promote relaxation. By reducing stress, meditation can help reduce the severity and frequency of ulcer symptoms.

Yoga

Yoga is another mind-body technique that can help heal stomach ulcers. Yoga involves a combination of meditation, breathing exercises, and physical postures. Several studies have shown that practicing yoga can help reduce stress, improve digestion, and decrease inflammation.

Regular yoga practice has been shown to reduce the severity of ulcer symptoms, such as pain, bloating, and nausea. In addition, yoga can help promote healing by increasing blood flow to the stomach and improving nutrient absorption.

Stress

Stress reduction techniques such as deep breathing, progressive muscle relaxation, and visualization can help heal stomach ulcers. Deep breathing exercises can help reduce stress and improve blood flow to the stomach, promoting healing.

Progressive muscle relaxation involves tensing and relaxing different muscle groups to promote relaxation and reduce stress.

Visualization techniques involve imagining a peaceful and calming scene to help minimize stress and anxiety.

Lifestyle Changes

In addition to these mind-body techniques, lifestyle changes can also help promote the healing of stomach ulcers. Avoiding alcohol, caffeine, and spicy foods can help reduce inflammation and irritation in the stomach.

A balanced diet with plenty of fruits, vegetables, and whole grains can also help reduce inflammation and promote healing. Sleeping, exercising regularly, and practicing good hygiene can also help reduce stress and promote healing.

In conclusion, mind-body techniques such as meditation, yoga, and stress reduction can play an essential role in healing stomach ulcers. These techniques can help reduce stress, promote relaxation, and improve digestion, which can all contribute to lowering ulcer symptoms and promoting healing.

While medical treatment is essential for ulcer healing, incorporating mind-body techniques into a comprehensive treatment plan can help improve overall health and well-being.

Chapter 5

Stomach Ulcer Healing and Prevention through Exercise and Physical Activity

Exercise and physical activity can be an essential part of the healing and prevention of stomach ulcers. When it comes to stomach ulcer healing and prevention, regular physical activity has several key benefits:

1. **Reduces stress:**

Chronic stress can contribute to ulcer formation and exacerbate the symptoms of existing ulcers. Exercise has been shown to reduce stress and improve mood, supporting the healing and prevention of stomach ulcers.

2. **Boosts the immune system:**

A strong immune system is essential for fighting off infections such as H. pylori, a leading cause of stomach ulcers. Exercise has been shown to boost the immune system and improve overall health.

3. **Improves digestion:**

Exercise can help improve digestion and reduce the risk of constipation, which can be beneficial for healing and preventing stomach ulcers.

4. *Increases blood flow:*

Exercise increases blood flow to the digestive system, which can help to support the healing process and reduce the risk of ulcer formation.

When it comes to incorporating exercise into your routine, the key is to find an activity that you enjoy and that fits into your lifestyle. Some options may include walking, running, swimming, yoga, pilates, strength training, or dancing. To increase your workouts' intensity and duration, start slowly and gradually increase your intensity and duration as you go.

It's also a good idea to consult with a healthcare professional before starting any new exercise program, especially if you have any pre-existing health conditions.

By making exercise and physical activity a regular part of your routine, you can support the healing and prevention of stomach ulcers and improve your overall health and well-being.

The Role of Exercise and Physical Activity in Stomach Ulcer Healing and Prevention

Exercise and physical activity can be an essential part of the healing and prevention of stomach ulcers. Regular physical activity has numerous health benefits, including reducing stress, boosting the immune system, and improving digestion. All of these factors can support the healing and prevention of stomach ulcers.

When it comes to exercise and physical activity, the key is to find an activity that you enjoy and that fits into your lifestyle. Some options may include the following:

- Walking or running

- Swimming or water aerobics

- Yoga or pilates

- Strength training

- Dancing

Increasing the intensity and duration of your workouts should be done slowly and gradually. It's also a good idea to consult with a healthcare professional before starting any new exercise program, especially if you have any pre-existing health conditions.

In addition to the physical benefits of exercise, it's also essential to consider the mental and emotional benefits. Exercise can help to reduce stress and improve mood, both of which can support the healing and prevention of stomach ulcers.

By incorporating regular exercise and physical activity into your routine, you can support the healing and prevention of stomach ulcers and improve your overall health and well-being.

The Role of Hydrotherapy in Stomach Ulcer Healing

Hydrotherapy, also known as water therapy or aquatic therapy, uses water for therapeutic purposes. It can be an effective treatment for various conditions, including stomach ulcers.

There are several ways that hydrotherapy can be used to support stomach ulcer healing:

1. **Reduces stress:**

Hydrotherapy has been shown to reduce stress and improve mood, which can benefit stomach ulcer healing. The warmth and buoyancy of the water can create a relaxing and soothing environment, which can help to reduce stress and promote healing.

2. *Improves circulation:*

Hydrotherapy can improve circulation and increase blood flow to the digestive system, which can help to support the healing process.

3. **Increases flexibility and range of motion:**

The buoyancy of the water can allow for a greater range of motion and help improve flexibility. Increasing flexibility and range of motion can benefit people experiencing pain or discomfort from stomach ulcers.

4. **Provides support and relief:**

The buoyancy of the water can help reduce pressure on the joints and muscles, providing support and relief for people with stomach ulcers.

Hydrotherapy can be performed in a pool, spa, or hot tub. It's essential to consult with a healthcare professional before starting a hydrotherapy program, especially if you have any pre-existing health conditions.

By incorporating hydrotherapy into your treatment plan, you can support the healing and prevention of stomach ulcers and improve your overall health and well-being.

Conventional Medical Treatments for Stomach Ulcers

Stomach ulcers, or peptic ulcers, are open sores that develop in the stomach lining or the small intestine. Various factors, including bacterial infections, prolonged use of certain medications, excessive alcohol consumption, and stress, can cause these ulcers. If left untreated, stomach ulcers can lead to severe complications such as bleeding, perforation, and obstruction.

Fortunately, there are several conventional medical treatments available for stomach ulcers. These treatments range from medications to procedures and aim to reduce inflammation, control acid secretion, and promote healing.

Medications

1. *Proton pump inhibitors (PPIs):*

PPIs are a class of medications that reduce the amount of acid the stomach produces. Examples of PPIs include pantoprazole, lansoprazole, and omeprazole. These medications are highly effective in promoting the healing of stomach ulcers and preventing recurrence.

2. *H2 receptor blockers:*

H2 receptor blockers are another class of medications that reduce the amount of acid produced by the stomach. Examples of H2 blockers include ranitidine, famotidine, and cimetidine. These medications are also effective in treating stomach ulcers but are less potent than PPIs.

3. Antacids:

Antacids are medications that neutralize stomach acid. Examples of antacids include calcium carbonate, magnesium hydroxide, and aluminum hydroxide. Antacids are often used in combination with other medications to provide immediate relief of symptoms.

4. Antibiotics:

Antibiotics treat stomach ulcers caused by bacterial infections, such as Helicobacter pylori (H. pylori). Examples of antibiotics used to treat H. pylori include amoxicillin, clarithromycin, and metronidazole.

Procedures

1. Endoscopy:

Endoscopy is a procedure that allows a gastroenterologist to view the inside of the stomach and the small intestine using a flexible tube with a camera attached to it. During the process, the doctor may take a biopsy (a small tissue sample) to check for H. pylori or other abnormalities.

2. **Surgery:**

Surgery is rarely needed to treat stomach ulcers, but it may be necessary in cases where the ulcer is bleeding or has perforated the stomach or small intestine. The damaged tissue is removed during surgery, and the area is repaired.

In conclusion, conventional medical treatments for stomach ulcers include a variety of medications and procedures. The treatment choice will depend on the ulcer's underlying cause, the symptoms' severity, and the complications' presence.

It is essential to seek medical attention if you experience stomach ulcer symptoms, as early diagnosis and treatment can prevent serious complications.

Chapter 6

The Role of Herbal Remedies in Stomach Ulcer Healing and Prevention

Herbal remedies are natural from plants and have been used for centuries to treat various health conditions, including stomach ulcers. While the effectiveness of herbal remedies may vary from person to person, they can be a safe and effective option for some people.

Some herbs that may be helpful in the healing and prevention of stomach ulcers include:

- **Licorice root:**

Licorice root has been used for centuries to treat digestive issues, including stomach ulcers. It may help to soothe the lining of the stomach and promote healing.

- **Slippery elm:**

Slippery elm is a tree native to North America and has been used for centuries to treat digestive issues. It may help to soothe the lining of the stomach and promote healing.

- **Marshmallow root:**

Marshmallow root is a plant native to Europe and has been used for centuries to treat digestive issues. It may help to soothe the lining of the stomach and promote healing.

- **Turmeric:**

Turmeric is a spice native to South Asia and known for its anti-inflammatory properties. It may also promote healing while reducing inflammation.

- **Ginger**:

Ginger is a spice native to Asia known for its digestive benefits. It can also reduce inflammation and promote healing.

It's important to note that the effectiveness of herbal remedies may vary from person to person, and it's always best to consult with a healthcare professional before starting any new treatment.

Stomach Ulcer Healing and Prevention through Acupuncture and Massage Therapy

Acupuncture and massage therapy have been alternative medicine practices for centuries to treat various health conditions, including stomach ulcers. While the effectiveness of acupuncture and massage therapy may vary from person to person, they can be a safe and effective option for some people.

Here's how acupuncture and massage therapy may be helpful in the healing and prevention of stomach ulcers:

- ***Reduces stress:***

Acupuncture and massage therapy can help reduce stress and improve mood, which can be beneficial for healing stomach ulcers. The relaxation and calm induced by these therapies can help to reduce stress and promote healing.

- ***Improves circulation:***

Acupuncture and massage therapy can improve circulation and increase blood flow to the digestive system, which can help to support the healing process.

- ***Reduces inflammation:***

Acupuncture and massage therapy can reduce inflammation in the body, which can benefit stomach ulcer healing.

- ***Provides support and relief:***

Massage therapy can help to reduce muscle tension and provide support and relief for people with stomach ulcers.

It's important to note that acupuncture and a trained and licensed professional should perform massage therapy. It's also a good idea to consult a healthcare professional before starting any new treatment.

By incorporating acupuncture and massage therapy into your treatment plan, you can support the healing and prevention of stomach ulcers and improve your overall health and well-being.

The Role of Mindfulness and Meditation in Stomach Ulcer Healing

Mindfulness and meditation are practices that involve focusing the mind on the present moment and can be helpful in the healing and prevention of stomach ulcers.

Here's how mindfulness and meditation can be beneficial for stomach ulcer healing:

1. ***Reduces stress:***

Mindfulness and meditation have been shown to reduce stress and improve mood, which can benefit stomach ulcer healing. The relaxation and calm induced by these practices can help to reduce stress and promote healing.

2. ***Improves digestion:***

Mindfulness and meditation can help improve digestion and reduce the risk of constipation, which can be beneficial for healing stomach ulcer.

3. *Increases self-awareness:*

Mindfulness and meditation can increase self-awareness and allow individuals to understand their thoughts and emotions better. Increasing self-awareness can be helpful in the healing process as it will enable individuals to identify and address any negative thought patterns or behaviors that may be contributing to their ulcer.

4. *Promotes relaxation:*

Mindfulness and meditation can help promote relaxation and reduce muscle tension, providing support and relief for people with stomach ulcers.

Practices such as seated meditation, walking meditation, and mindful breathing all fall under the category of mindfulness and meditation. Trying other methods to see what works best for you is a good idea. Remembering to practice mindfulness and meditation in a safe and comfortable environment is also essential.

By incorporating mindfulness and meditation into your treatment plan, you can support the healing and prevention of stomach ulcers and improve your overall health and well-being.

Managing Stomach Ulcers in Children and Adolescents

Stomach ulcers, or peptic ulcers, are open sores that develop in the stomach lining or small intestine. Although stomach ulcers are more common in adults, they can also affect children and adolescents. Studies have shown that up to 10% of children and adolescents may eventually develop stomach ulcers.

Managing stomach ulcers in children and adolescents requires a careful approach considering the child's age, medical history, and symptoms.

Symptoms of Stomach Ulcers in Children and Adolescents:

The symptoms of stomach ulcers in children and adolescents are similar to those in adults and may include the following:

- Abdominal pain, which may be severe or mild

- Nausea and vomiting

- Loss of appetite

- Weight loss

- Fatigue

- Difficulty sleeping

Managing Stomach Ulcers in Children and Adolescents:

1. Medications:

The primary treatment for stomach ulcers in children and adolescents is medication. The most commonly used drugs include proton pump inhibitors (PPIs), H2 receptor blockers, and antacids.

These medications work by reducing the amount of acid the stomach produces, which can help relieve pain and promote healing. The medication dosage will depend on the child's age, weight, and medical history.

2. Dietary Changes:

In addition to medication, dietary changes may be recommended to manage stomach ulcers in children and adolescents. The child may be advised to eat smaller, more frequent meals and avoid spicy, acidic, or fatty foods that can irritate the stomach.

Additionally, the child may be encouraged to drink plenty of fluids and avoid caffeine and carbonated drinks.

3. *Stress Reduction:*

Stress can exacerbate stomach ulcers in children and adolescents. Therefore, I recommend stress reduction techniques such as relaxation exercises and counseling to help manage symptoms.

4. *Treatment of H. pylori Infection:*

If an H. pylori infection causes a stomach ulcer, the child must be treated with antibiotics and acid-suppressing medication. The treatment will usually last for two weeks, followed by a monitoring period to ensure the infection has been eradicated.

5. *Endoscopy*:

Most experts recommend endoscopy for children and adolescents with persistent or severe symptoms or if there is a suspicion of complications such as bleeding or perforation. During the procedure, a tiny camera is inserted through the mouth and into the stomach to examine the lining of the stomach and small intestine.

Bottom Line:

You can effectively manage stomach ulcers in children and adolescents with medications, dietary changes, stress reduction, and treatment of underlying infections. Working closely with a healthcare provider to develop a treatment plan appropriate for the child's age, medical history, and symptoms are essential.

With proper management, most children and adolescents with stomach ulcers will fully recover and experience no long-term complications.

Chapter 7

The Role of Nutrition in Stomach Ulcer Healing and Prevention

Proper nutrition is an integral part of healing and preventing stomach ulcers. Eating a healthy, balanced diet can support the healing process and reduce your risk of ulcer formation.

Here are some tips for healthy eating during the stomach ulcer healing process:

1. ***Eat a variety of fruits and vegetables:***

Fruits and vegetables are rich in antioxidants, which can help to reduce inflammation and support the healing process. Try going for at least five servings of vegetables and fruits per day.

2. ***Choose whole grains:***

Whole grains are a good source of fiber, which can help to improve digestion and reduce the risk of constipation. Choose whole-grain rice, pasta, and bread instead of refined grains.

3. ***Include lean proteins:***

Lean proteins, such as chicken, fish, and tofu, can help to support the healing process. Choose lean proteins and limit your intake of red meat.

4. ***Avoid spicy and acidic foods:***

Spicy and acidic foods can irritate the lining of the stomach and exacerbate the symptoms of ulcers. Avoid spicy and acidic foods and opt for milder options instead.

5. ***Limit alcohol and caffeine:***

Excessive consumption of alcohol and caffeine can irritate the lining of the stomach and increase the risk of ulcer formation. Limit your intake of these substances and choose non-caffeinated beverages instead.

Following a healthy, balanced diet can support the healing and prevention of stomach ulcers and improve your overall health and well-being.

Stomach Ulcer Healing and Prevention through Yoga and Breathwork

Yoga and breathwork are practices that involve physical postures and controlled breathing techniques and can be helpful in the healing and prevention of stomach ulcers.

Here's how yoga and breathwork can be beneficial for stomach ulcer healing:

1. *Reduces stress:*

Yoga and breathwork have been shown to reduce stress and improve mood, which can benefit stomach ulcer healing. The relaxation and calm induced by these practices can help to reduce stress and promote healing.

2. *Improves digestion:*

Yoga and breathwork can help improve digestion and reduce the risk of constipation, which can be beneficial for healing stomach ulcers.

3. *Increases self-awareness:*

Yoga and breathwork can increase self-awareness and allow individuals to understand their thoughts and emotions better. Increasing self-awareness can be helpful in the healing process as it will enable individuals to identify and address any negative thought patterns or behaviors that may be contributing to their ulcer.

4. *Promotes relaxation:*

Yoga and breathwork can help promote relaxation and reduce muscle tension, providing support and relief for people with stomach ulcers.

There are many different types of yoga and breathwork practices, and it's a good idea to try other techniques to see what works best for you. Practising yoga and breathwork in a safe and comfortable environment and consulting with a healthcare professional before starting any new program are essential.

By incorporating yoga and breathwork into your treatment plan, you can support the healing and prevention of stomach ulcers and improve your overall health and well-being.

The Role of Essential Oils in Stomach Ulcer Healing and Prevention

Essential oils are natural oils extracted from plants and have been used for centuries in traditional medicine to treat various health conditions, including stomach ulcers. While the effectiveness of essential oils may vary from person to person, they can be a safe and effective option for some people.

Here's how essential oils may be helpful in the healing and prevention of stomach ulcers:

1. **Reduces stress:**

Essential oils, such as lavender and chamomile, have been shown to reduce stress and improve mood, which can be beneficial for stomach ulcer healing. The relaxation and calm induced by these oils can help to reduce stress and promote healing.

2. *Reduces inflammation:*

Essential oils, such as turmeric and ginger, have anti-inflammatory properties and can help reduce inflammation in the body, which can be beneficial for healing stomach ulcers.

3. *Improves digestion:*

Essential oils, such as peppermint and fennel, can help improve digestion and reduce the risk of constipation, which can be beneficial for healing stomach ulcers.

4. *Provides support and relief:*

Essential oils, such as frankincense and myrrh, can help to reduce muscle tension and provide support and relief for people with stomach ulcers.

It's important to note that essential oils should be used cautiously and diluted with carrier oil before use. It's also a good idea to consult a healthcare professional before starting any new treatment.

By incorporating essential oils into your treatment plan, you can support the healing and prevention of stomach ulcers and improve your overall health and well-being.

Lifestyle Changes for Stomach Ulcer Prevention and Maintenance

Stomach ulcers, or gastric ulcers, are painful sores that develop in the stomach lining. Various factors, including stress, bacterial infections, and certain medications, can cause them.

If left untreated, stomach ulcers can lead to severe complications such as bleeding and perforation of the stomach wall. However, there are several lifestyle changes that individuals can make to prevent and manage stomach ulcers.

1. *Adopt a healthy diet:*

A balanced and healthy diet is crucial for preventing and managing stomach ulcers. Adopting a healthy diet means consuming a diet rich in fruits, vegetables, lean proteins, and whole grains. Avoiding spicy, acidic, and greasy foods can also help to reduce the risk of developing stomach ulcers.

Additionally, individuals should aim to eat smaller, more frequent meals throughout the day to help manage symptoms.

2. *Manage stress:*

Stress is a common trigger for stomach ulcers. Therefore, individuals should adopt stress management techniques such as yoga, meditation, or deep breathing exercises. Regular exercise can also improve overall health and help to reduce stress.

3. **Avoid smoking and excessive alcohol consumption:**

Smoking and excessive alcohol consumption can irritate the stomach lining and increase the risk of developing stomach ulcers. Individuals who smoke should consider quitting, while those who drink alcohol should do so in moderation.

4. **Take medication as prescribed:**

Some medications can increase the risk of developing stomach ulcers. Therefore, individuals should only take medication as prescribed by their healthcare provider.

Additionally, individuals should inform their healthcare provider if they experience stomach pain or discomfort while taking medication.

5. **Practice good hygiene:**

Stomach ulcers can be caused by bacterial infections such as Helicobacter pylori. Therefore, individuals should practice good hygiene by washing their hands regularly and avoiding sharing utensils or drinking glasses with others.

6. **Get regular check-ups:**

Regular check-ups with a healthcare provider can help to identify and manage stomach ulcers. During a check-up, a healthcare provider may perform tests to check for bacterial infections or other underlying conditions that may increase the risk of developing stomach ulcers.

In conclusion, adopting a healthy lifestyle can go a long way in preventing and managing stomach ulcers. A balanced diet, stress management techniques, avoiding smoking and excessive alcohol consumption, taking medication as prescribed, practicing good hygiene, and regular check-ups with a healthcare provider are all crucial for maintaining good digestive health.

Individuals who experience stomach pain or discomfort should seek medical attention as soon as possible to receive prompt diagnosis and treatment.

Chapter 8

The Role of Stress Management in Stomach Ulcer Healing and Prevention

Stress is a normal part of life, but chronic stress can negatively impact our health, including increasing the risk of ulcer formation and exacerbating the symptoms of existing ulcers. Therefore, it's important to practice stress management techniques to support the healing and prevention of stomach ulcers.

Here are some tips for managing stress:

- **Practice relaxation techniques**: Techniques such as deep breathing, meditation, and yoga can help to reduce stress and improve mood.

- **Exercise regularly**: Exercise has been shown to reduce stress and improve mood. Choose an activity you enjoy and make it a routine.

- **Get enough sleep**: Adequate sleep is vital for overall health and can help to reduce stress. Aim for 7-9 hours of sleep per night.

- **Eat a healthy diet**: A healthy, balanced diet can support overall health and reduce stress. Choose whole, unprocessed foods and limit your intake of alcohol and caffeine.

- **Seek support**: It can be helpful to talk to a trusted friend or family member about your stress or to seek the support of a mental health professional.

By practicing stress management techniques, you can support the healing and prevention of stomach ulcers and improve your overall health and well-being.

Stomach Ulcer Healing and Prevention through Homeopathy

Homeopathy is a system of alternative medicine that involves using small doses of natural substances to stimulate the body's healing process. Homeopathy may be helpful in the healing and prevention of stomach ulcers.

Here's how homeopathy may be beneficial for stomach ulcer healing:

1. *Reduces stress:*

Homeopathic remedies, such as Ignatia and Natrum muriaticum, have been shown to reduce stress and improve mood, benefiting stomach ulcer healing. The relaxation and calm induced by these remedies can help to reduce stress and promote healing.

2. *Improves digestion:*

Homeopathic remedies, such as Nux vomica and Arsenicum album, can help improve digestion and reduce the risk of constipation, which can be beneficial for healing stomach ulcers.

3. *Reduces inflammation:*

Homeopathic remedies, such as Belladonna and Bryonia, have anti-inflammatory properties and can help reduce inflammation in the body, which can be beneficial for healing stomach ulcers.

4. *Provides support and relief:*

Homeopathic remedies, such as Phosphorus and Carbo vegetabilis, can help to reduce muscle tension and provide support and relief for people with stomach ulcers.

It's important to note that you can use homeopathic remedies with caution and under the guidance of a trained and licensed homeopath. It's also a good idea to consult a healthcare professional before starting any new treatment.

By incorporating homeopathy into your treatment plan, you can support the healing and prevention of stomach ulcers and improve your overall health and well-being.

Integrating Natural Remedies into Your Stomach Ulcer Healing Plan

Incorporating natural remedies into your stomach ulcer healing plan can be a safe and effective way to support healing and reduce the risk of ulcer formation. Many natural remedies can be helpful, including herbal remedies, acupuncture, massage therapy, mindfulness and meditation, nutrition, yoga and breathwork, essential oils, and homeopathy.

Here are some tips for integrating natural remedies into your stomach ulcer healing plan:

1. ***Consult with a healthcare professional:***

It's always a good idea to consult a healthcare professional before starting any new treatment, including natural remedies. A healthcare professional can help you determine the best treatment for your specific needs and ensure that any natural remedies you consider are safe and appropriate.

2. ***Choose high-quality products:***

When choosing natural remedies, it's essential to select products from reputable manufacturers and to carefully read labels to ensure that you are using the product correctly.

3. **Consider the potential risks and benefits:**

While natural remedies can be effective, it's essential to consider each treatment's potential risks and benefits before starting. Some natural remedies may interact with medications you are taking or may have side-effects you should be aware of.

4. **Be consistent:**

You must be consistent with your natural remedies and use them as directed to see the best results.

Integrating natural remedies into your stomach ulcer healing plan and working closely with a healthcare professional can support the healing process and improve your overall health and well-being.

The Future of Stomach Ulcer Treatment

Stomach ulcers, also known as gastric ulcers, are a common condition affecting millions worldwide. While several effective treatments are available for stomach ulcers, including antibiotics, acid-suppressing medications, and lifestyle changes, researchers continue to explore new therapies that may provide even better patient outcomes.

This section will explore some emerging therapies and research related to the future of stomach ulcer treatment.

1. Probiotics:

Probiotics are living microorganisms that are believed to have health benefits when consumed. Recent research has suggested that certain probiotic strains may help prevent and treat stomach ulcers by improving the balance of bacteria in the digestive system.

However, more research is needed to determine the effectiveness of probiotics for treating stomach ulcers.

2. *Stem cell therapy:*

Stem cell therapy involves using stem cells to repair damaged tissues and promote healing. Researchers are exploring the potential of stem cell therapy for treating stomach ulcers, with early studies suggesting that it may effectively reduce ulcer size and promote healing.

However, more research is needed to determine the safety and effectiveness of stem cell therapy for stomach ulcers.

3. *Gene therapy:*

Gene therapy involves the use of genetic material to treat or prevent disease. Researchers are exploring the potential of gene therapy for treating stomach ulcers by targeting genes involved in the development of ulcers.

While still in the early stages of research, gene therapy may hold promise as a future treatment option for stomach ulcers.

4. Nanoparticle therapy:

Nanoparticle therapy involves using tiny particles to deliver drugs or other treatments directly to the site of the ulcer. Researchers are exploring the potential of nanoparticle therapy for treating stomach ulcers, with early studies suggesting that it may be an effective way to deliver drugs and promote healing.

5. Herbal and natural remedies:

Herbal and natural remedies, such as honey, licorice root, and aloe vera, have been used for centuries to treat digestive disorders, including stomach ulcers. Researchers are exploring the potential of these remedies for treating stomach ulcers, with some studies suggesting that they may effectively reduce ulcer size and promote healing.

However, more research is needed to determine the safety and effectiveness of these remedies.

In conclusion, while several effective treatments are available for stomach ulcers, researchers continue to explore new therapies and approaches that may provide even better patient outcomes.

From probiotics and stem cell therapy to gene therapy and nanoparticle therapy, there are many exciting avenues for future research and development in the field of stomach ulcer treatment.

As research continues to advance, patients with stomach ulcers can look forward to improved treatments and outcomes.

Conclusion

In conclusion, "*The Natural Way to Heal Stomach Ulcers*" has explored a variety of natural remedies and lifestyle changes that can be helpful in the healing and prevention of stomach ulcers. There are many different options, from herbal remedies and acupuncture to mindfulness and meditation, nutrition, and yoga and breathwork.

It's important to remember that the effectiveness of natural remedies may vary from person to person, and it's always a good idea to consult with a healthcare professional before starting any new treatment.

By integrating natural remedies into your treatment plan and working closely with a healthcare professional, you can support the healing and prevention of stomach ulcers and improve your overall health and well-being.

I hope this book has provided you with the information and resources you need to relieve the pain and discomfort of stomach ulcers and take control of your health. We wish you the best on your journey to healing and lasting relief.

Epilogue

As we end this book, I hope the strategies outlined within its pages have been a source of hope and healing for those suffering from stomach ulcers. Throughout these chapters, we have explored the many natural approaches to healing that can provide lasting relief from the pain and discomfort associated with this condition.

We have discussed the importance of a healthy diet and lifestyle, including probiotics, fiber, and other vital nutrients, in promoting gut health. We have also examined the benefits of herbal remedies and natural supplements, such as licorice root and aloe vera, which can help to reduce inflammation and promote healing in the digestive tract.

Above all, we have emphasized the importance of a holistic approach to healing that recognizes the interconnectedness of mind, body, and spirit. By reducing stress, practicing mindfulness, and cultivating a positive mindset, we can support our body's natural healing processes and promote lasting relief from stomach ulcers.

Of course, every individual's journey to healing is unique, and there may be challenges along the way. But I encourage you to remain steadfast in your commitment to natural healing and draw upon the many resources available, including healthcare professionals, support groups, and alternative practitioners.

Ultimately, the path to healing is a journey that requires patience, persistence, and self-care. But with the right tools and strategies in place, it is a journey that can lead to lasting relief, renewed vitality, and a profound sense of well-being. May this book be a valuable resource on your path to healing, and may you find the peace and comfort you deserve.

About the Author

Kayla S. Brigman is a natural health practitioner with over 16 years of experience helping people achieves optimal health and wellness. She has a deep passion for holistic medicine and believes in the power of natural remedies to heal the body and mind.

In her practice, Kayla has helped countless patients suffering from stomach ulcers by providing natural, effective treatments that address the root causes of their symptoms. She has a wealth of knowledge on the latest scientific research and techniques in the field of natural medicine and is dedicated to sharing this information with others.

Kayla S. Brigman is also a renowned speaker and educator, having presented at numerous conferences and seminars on topics such as natural remedies for digestive health, stress management, and holistic healing. She is a regular contributor to health and wellness publications and has been featured in various media outlets for her expertise in natural health.

With "*The Natural Way to Heal Stomach Ulcers*," Kayla shares her knowledge and insights on how to alleviate the symptoms of stomach ulcers using natural remedies and proven techniques. She believes that healing the body naturally is not only effective but can also be a transformative and empowering experience for individuals seeking to take control of their health.

Other Books by the Author

Below are other amazing book(s) by Kayla S. Brigman

BOOK TITLE	BOOK COVER	LINK TO READ
End The Snore Struggle		Click Here to read for free on Kindle Unlimited
The Art of Being Fresh		Click Here to read for free on Kindle Unlimited

The Lean Body Blueprint		[Click Here to read for free on Kindle Unlimited](#)
Postpartum Body Rejuvenation For Women		[Click Here to read for free on Kindle Unlimited](#)
Kiss Bad Breath Goodbye		[Click Here to read for free on Kindle Unlimited](#)

The Anti-Aging Blueprint	THE ANTI-AGING BLUEPRINT KAYLA S. BRIGMAN	<u>Click Here to read for free on Kindle Unlimited</u>
Going Bald with Grace	GOING BALD WITH GRACE Embracing and Empowering Yourself after Hair Loss KAYLA S. BRIGMAN	<u>Click Here to read for free on Kindle Unlimited</u>
The Flat Tummy Blueprint	THE FLAT TUMMY BLUEPRINT Simple Strategies for a Leaner Midsection KAYLA S. BRIGMAN	<u>Click Here to read for free on Kindle Unlimited</u>

THE END